This Journal Belongs to

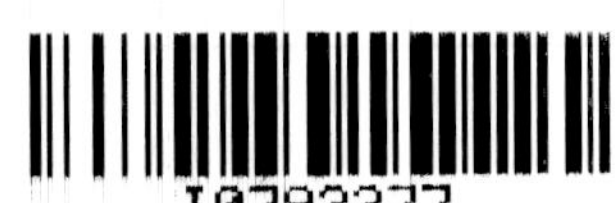

My Mission Statement

My Journey Starts On